T0368489

Twinkle, Twinkle, Little Finkle

AuthorHouse™
1663 Liberty Drive
Bloomington, IN 47403
www.authorhouse.com
Phone: 833-262-8899

This book is printed on acid-free paper.

ISBN: 979-8-8230-1798-5 (sc)
ISBN: 979-8-8230-1799-2 (hc)
ISBN: 979-8-8230-1800-5 (e)

Library of Congress Control Number: 2023922000

Print information available on the last page.

Published by AuthorHouse 01/02/2023

author HOUSE®

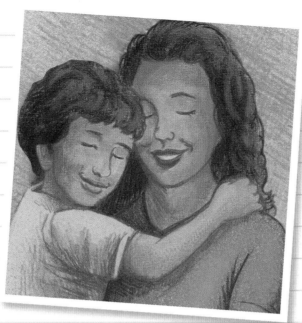

Twinkle, Twinkle, Little Finkle

By James D. Waedekin

Illustrations by Dan Drewes

On the day Raymond is born, Mrs. Finkle thinks the world is divine. Picture-perfect in Daddy's hands, she knows his twinkle will surely shine.

Like his brothers, he glows, laughs and cries. Like his sisters, he glimmers, burps and sighs.

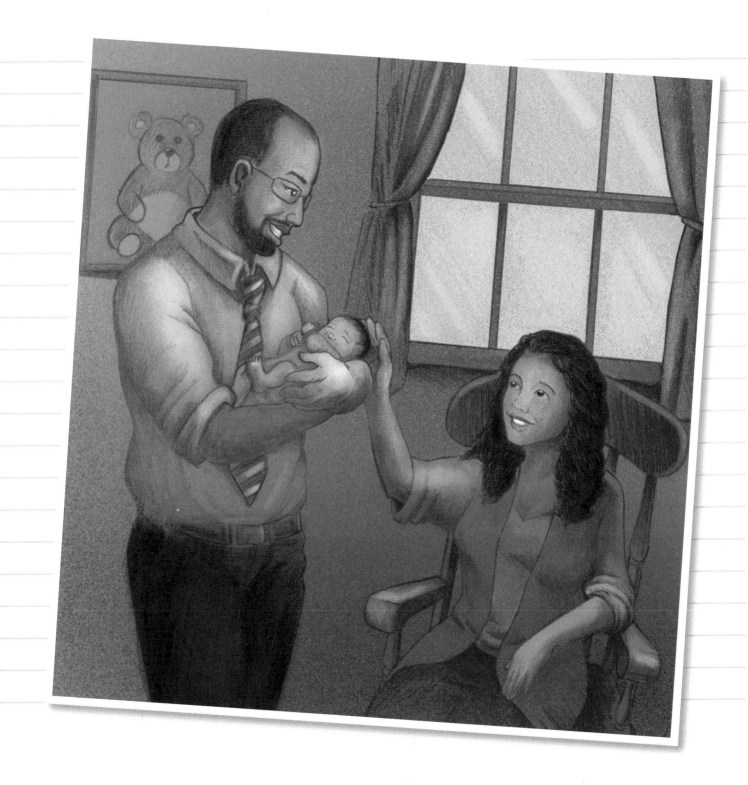

But alas, unlike the many Finkles before him, his journey looks somewhat bleak. Although he grows taller like the neighborhood toddlers ...

... Raymond will not speak.

3

Afraid for their son, the Finkles have Raymond's hearing checked. The ear doctor sends the bill and note:

"NORMAL.
TESTS ALWAYS CORRECT."

Afraid for their son, the Finkles have Raymond's eyesight verified. The eye doctor sends the bill and note:

"NORMAL.
DON'T BE TERRIFIED."

4

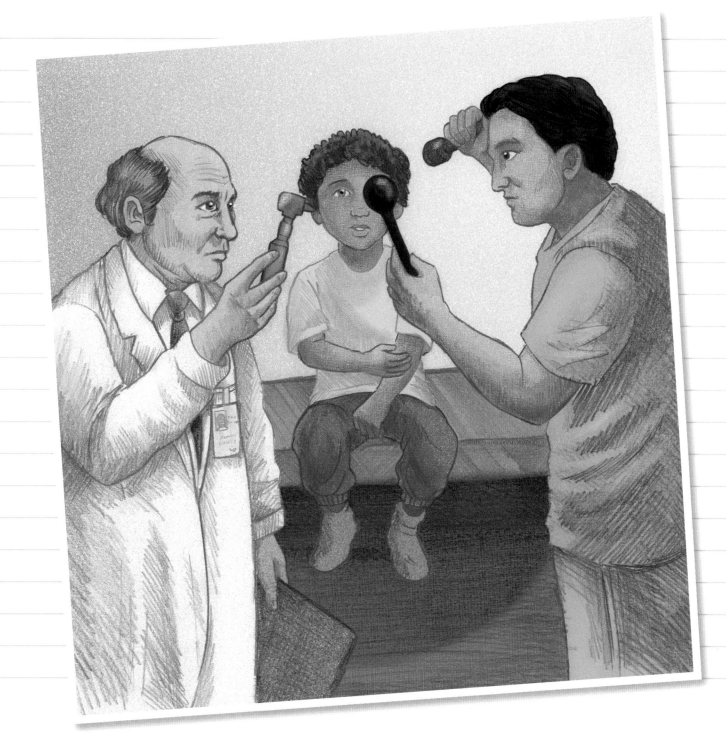

Mrs. Finkle thinks ...

"If Little Ray can hear, and Little Ray can see ... then why won't he speak like the other Finkles, even a little bit ... just for me?"

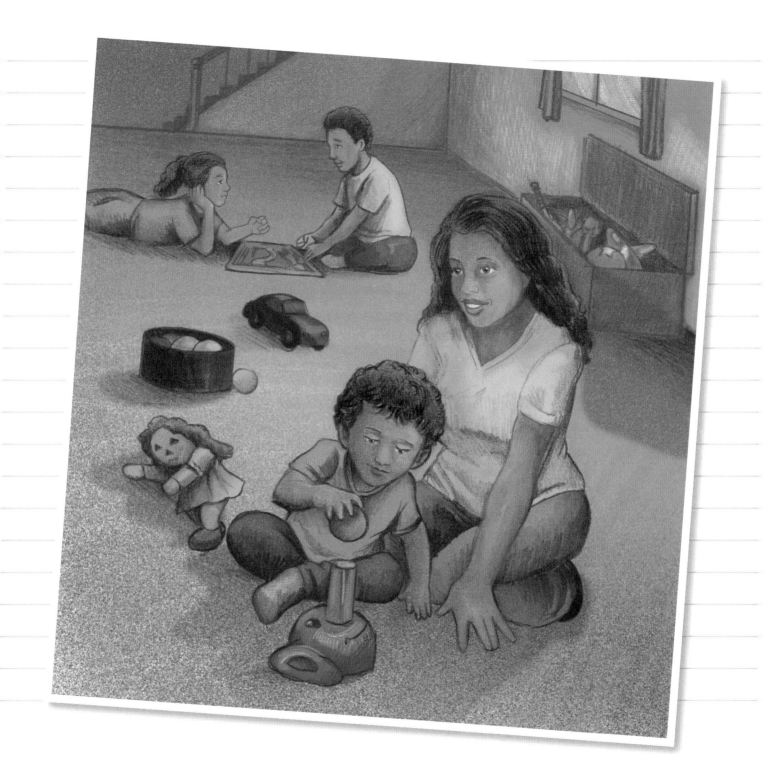

"It's quite simple," Mr. Spencer the Specialist confounds, compounding Mr. & Mrs. Finkle's fears. "Your little Raymond Finkle is COM--MUN--I--CA--TIVE--LY wrinkled!" And the Finkles fight back tears. "Do not fear. Trust me, I promise, this disorder soon shall pass. These phases are a bother, but rarely ever last!"

As Raymond grows taller, this "neverlasting soonly passing" spell hurts his schoolwork, and his little spirit too. He falls fast behind his classmates' skills and the lessons his teacher Miss Jones assigns for him to do.

If they do not get Little Ray some help, their son could fade before their eyes, so onward the Finkles search for answers from the SPEAKING WORLD's wise.

"Articulation ... Fluency ... Voice ..."
the clever counselors croon.

"Articulation ... Fluency ... Voice ..."
more trusty therapists tune.

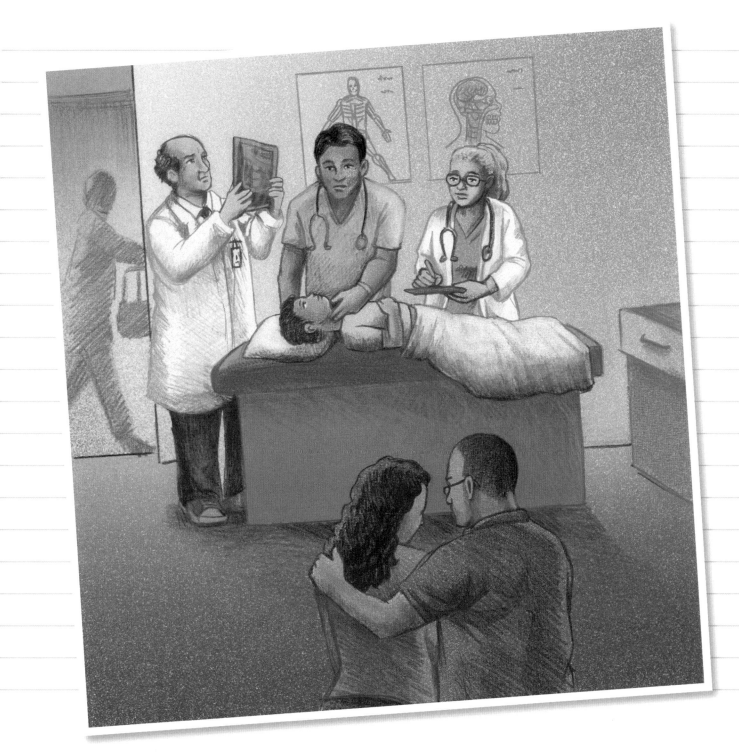

ARTICULATION

"He'll grow out of it ... articulate soooooo nice," Dr. Clearup pronounces slowly and precise. "Many sons and daughters, during younger years, exhibit this difficult song. My intensive speech training, both rigorous and draining, will have him talking before long."

FLUENCY

"I can't even understand a word
Raymond whispers," Dr. Gurgle slurs,
(wishing his OWN voice was crisper).
"WHO hit him in the head and damaged
his brain? WHICH of his parents make
Raymond feel blame?

Is it PHYSIOLOGICAL (body)
or PSYCHOLOGICAL (mind)?

We NEVER will know. But Raymond's
fluency problem has got to get and go!"

VOICE

"Raymond's voice is just dandy and fine," Dr. Drag tones with an irritating whine, "His vocal cords are not damaged. Don't appear strained. His breathing is very clear so allergies won't be blamed. His quick Finkle mind and quick Finkle lips form simply solid sounds. A few lessons with me and his shouts will soar way, way out of bounds!"

To make matters worse, every day at school, the silent Raymond fits a label. Rarely talks. When he does ... trips over his tongue. The other kids think he's unstable!

"Go on! We're waiting! For words! Spit them out!"

Stinky mean bullies point fingers and shout.

"We d-d-d-don't got all day," children meanly sputter.

"Not all day for you to STU-U-U-T-TER!"

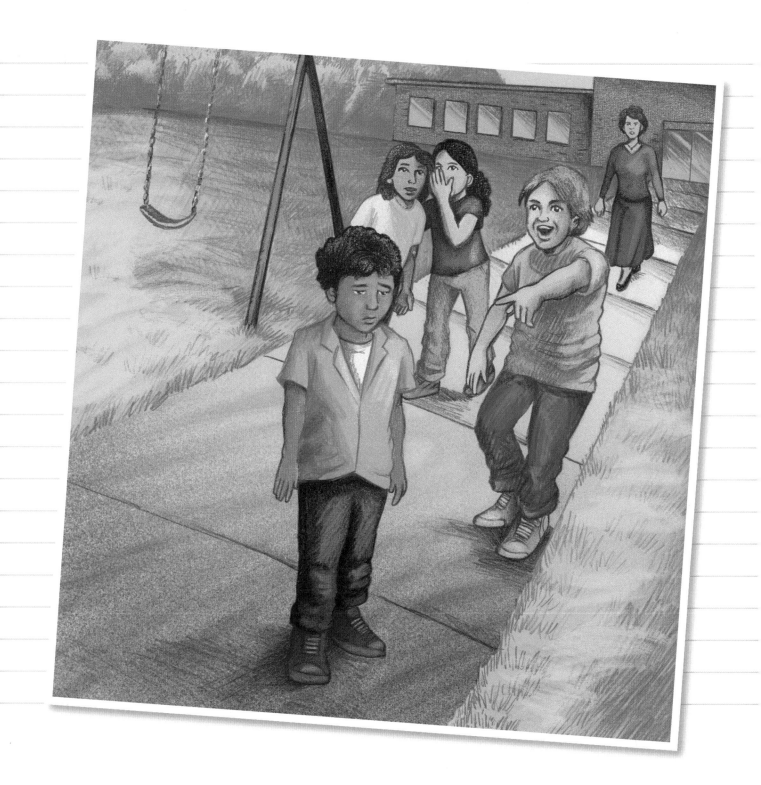

MORE often than not Raymond shuts
down. He stands quiet, alone and always
frowns. WHERE will he find the support
he needs? Families and friends and
teachers take heed. EVERYONE around
him corrects his words or never waits
for Raymond to be heard. AND people
are always impatient, and interrupt his
thoughts, UNTIL his head is full of
pressure and really big brain clots.

17

"Won't someone take the time to really listen?" Raymond says to the mirror in his room. His words NEVER topple or tumble … the mirror smiles back at his fine tune.

For words from his mouth flow easy and free … when it is just him … with no one to see.

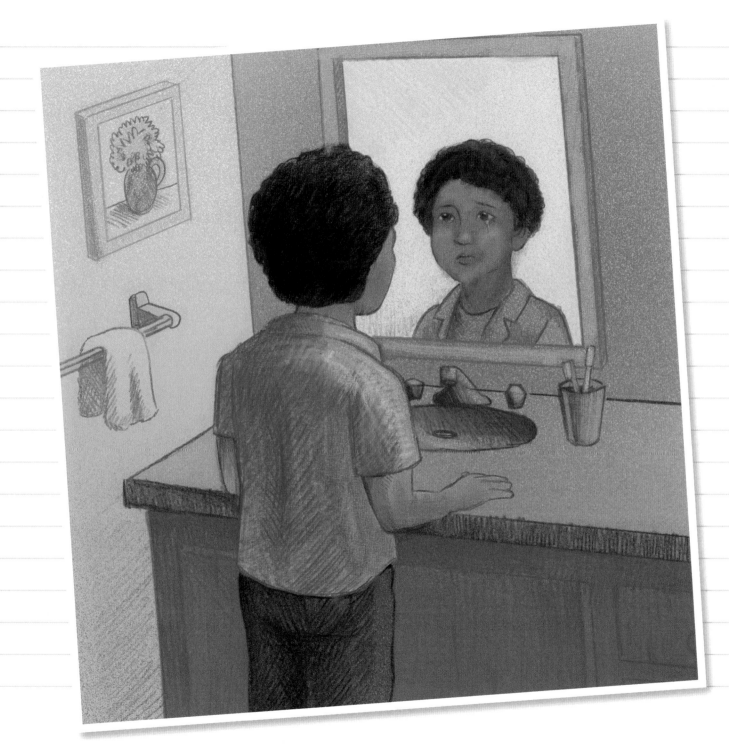

Day after day Little Ray whispers his wishes, ever so quietly though no one listens:

WISH #1

"Maybe those around me could somehow help, and quit their mean barking and hateful yelps."

WISH #2

"Maybe good listeners would take more time, so they would know I too can rhyme."

WISH #3

"Maybe good teachers could present their lessons with simple steps so I could join in with right answers, hear cheers and grow pep."

WISH #4

"Wouldn't it be nice... if everyone modeled good language skills too? I could learn from them by listening, not feeling so blue."

WISH #5

"What if teachers and students and family alike, would elaborate on my words, help me feel bright? Then I could add to my mind night after night, the words right now that give me a fright."

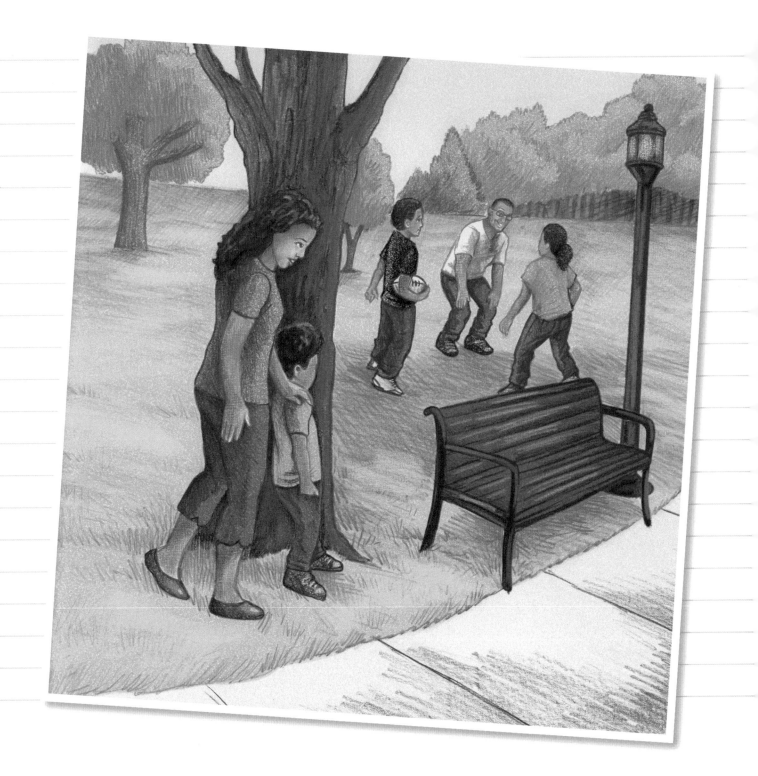

The Finkles still hope when the timing is just right, perfect speech will sprout from their youngest of sprites. Hushed chuckles and whispers might grow to cheers, as all around will someday hear ... the words from this Finkle with something to say. They know in their hearts he will not fade away.

Finally, one spring afternoon as the very merry last school bell rings, boys and girls from all over corner Raymond at the playground swings.

"Go on! We're waiting! For words! Spit 'em out!"

Stinky mean bullies point fingers and shout.

"We d-d-d-don't got all day," children meanly sputter.

"Not all day for you to STU-U-U-T-TER!"

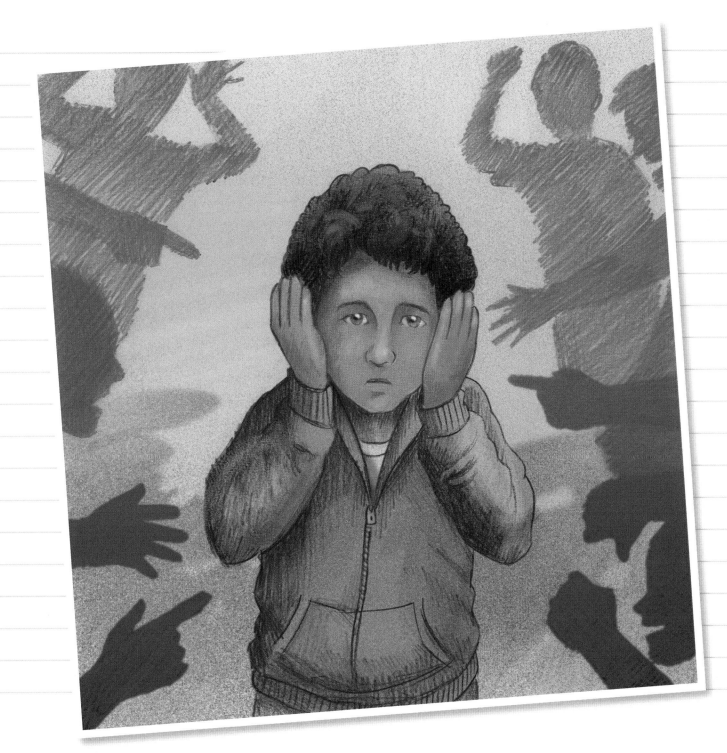

But this day is different, Raymond feels
something new inside, he no longer
runs or backs down ... and refuses to
hide.

As Raymond consumes a deep breath
they gasp, and their pools of laughter
halt suddenly fast. So with the greatest
of ease, like a gentle cool breeze,
Raymond simply says at last:

"Maybe I don't want to talk. Maybe you're not worth my time. You all should be ashamed of yourselves and your crime ....

... All these years I had something to say, and you were my burden, got in my way ....

... I may speak slow, sometimes putter and stutter, but my mind races with thoughts which fly and flutter!

... And if you're lucky, maybe someday I'll share with you ...What wonders true speech and language can do!"

31

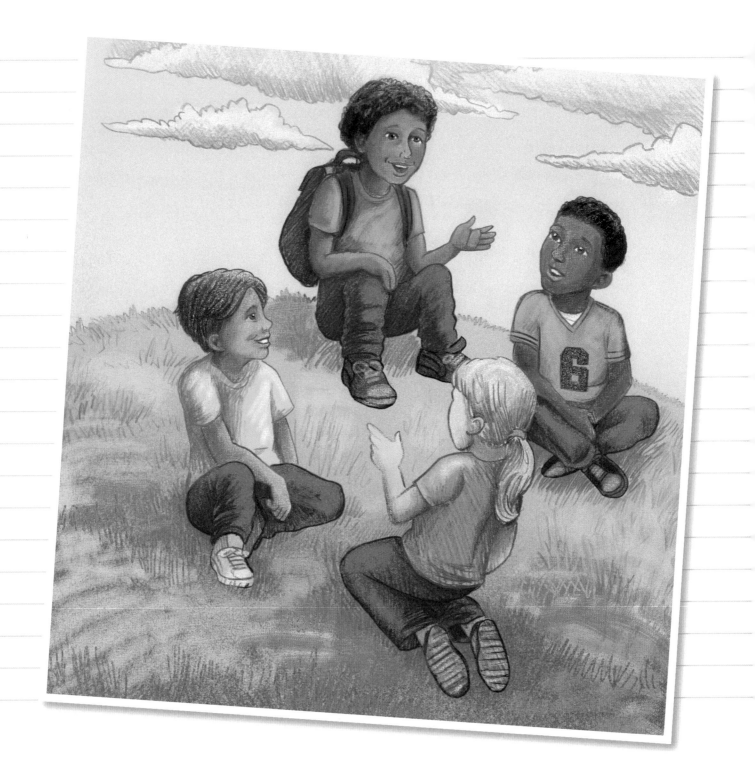

Stunned by his own words, before anyone has the faintest boldness to reply, Raymond turns and runs home, calling back his "Bye!" and "Good-byes!"

He slams the Finkle front door, jumping into his parents' warm arms. Upward he leaps ... free from the reach ... of a world's quite bitter harm.

His cheek against his mother's, where he always finds love, Raymond says ... ab-so-lute-ly nothing ... which the Finkles are proud of.

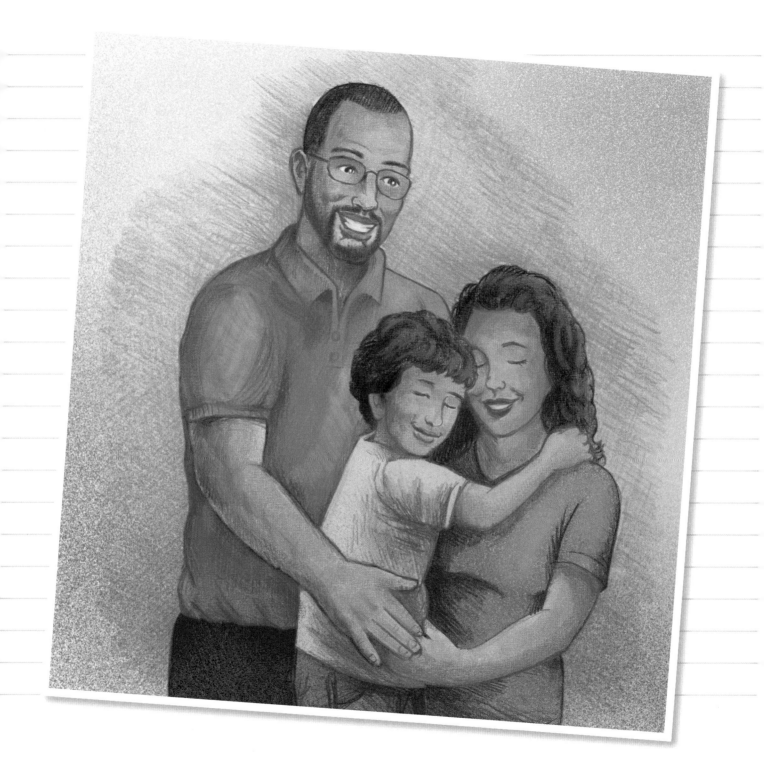

"How can this be?" each of you quickly asks me. "Surely he should share what he just said?" As my tale comes to an end, it's safe to say ... parents truly know what's in their child's head.

A hug is enough for our speechless Mr. & Mrs. Finkle.

At last. Yes, at last! Their hearts feel ...

Little Raymond's

growing

twinkle.

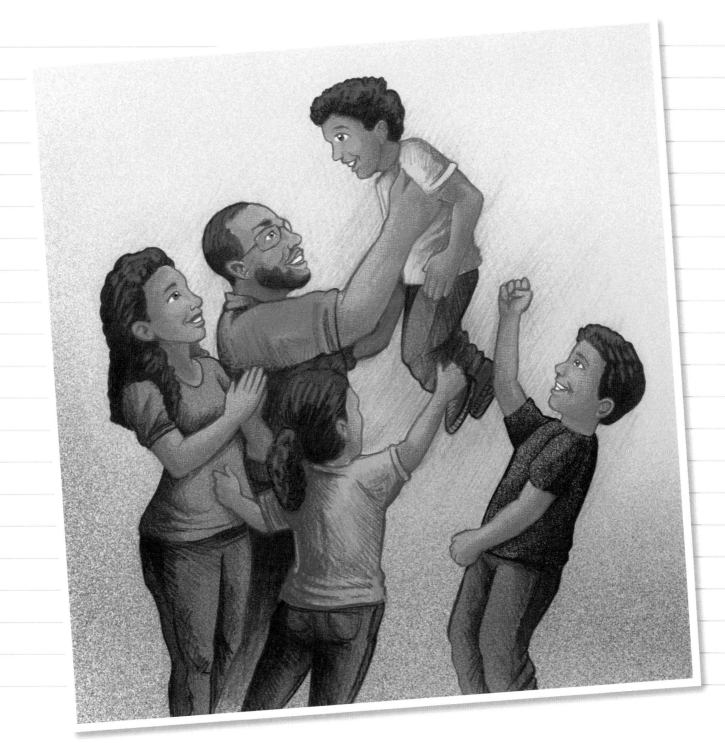

THE END

Printed in the United States
by Baker & Taylor Publisher Services